CANCER IS NOT GE

NATURAL SOLUTIONS TO OPTIMAL HEALTH

DR JOHN BERGMAN

Get the Truth below:

http://ic.instantcustomer.com/go/94500/lead-page-12350

WHY I WROTE THIS BOOK

I wrote this book because I am sick and tired of the mis-information that is so prevalent in America today. We spend the most on healthcare costs, so we assume that makes us the healthiest country in the world. The World Health Organization has come out with their latest rankings of the healthcare worldwide. A snapshot of those rankings is below.

World Health Organization Ranking; The World's Health Systems		
1 France	65 Uruguay	128 Guyana
2 Italy	66 Hungary	129 Peru
3 San Marino	67 Trinidad and Tobago	130 Russia
4 Andorra	68 Saint Lucia	131 Honduras
5 Malta	69 Belize	132 Burkina Faso
6 Singapore	70 Turkey	133 Sao Tome and Principe
7 Spain	71 Nicaragua	134 Sudan
8 Oman	72 Belarus	135 Ghana
9 Austria	73 Lithuania	136 Tuvalu
10 Japan	74 Saint Vincent and the Grenadines	137 Ivory Coast
11 Norway	75 Argentina	138 Haiti
12 Portugal	76 Sri Lanka	139 Gabon
13 Monaco	77 Estonia	140 Kenya
14 Greece	78 Guatemala	141 Marshall Islands
15 Iceland	79 Ukraine	142 Kiribati
16 Luxembourg	80 Solomon Islands	143 Burundi
17 Netherlands	81 Algeria	144 China
18 United Kingdom	82 Palau	145 Mongolia
19 Ireland	83 Jordan	146 Gambia
20 Switzerland	84 Mauritius	147 Maldives
21 Belgium	85 Grenada	148 Papua New Guinea
22 Colombia	86 Antigua and Barbuda	149 Uganda
23 Sweden	87 Libya	150 Nepal
24 Cyprus	88 Bangladesh	151 Kyrgystan
25 Germany	89 Macedonia	152 Togo
26 Saudi Arabia	90 Bosnia-Herzegovina	153 Turkmenistan
27 United Arab Emirates	91 Lebanon	154 Tajikistan
28 Israel	92 Indonesia	155 Zimbabwe
29 Morocco	93 Iran	156 Tanzania
30 Canada	94 Bahamas	157 Djibouti
31 Finland	95 Panama	158 Eritrea
32 Australia	96 Fiji	159 Madagascar
33 Chile	97 Benin	160 Vietnam
34 Denmark	98 Nauru	161 Guinea
35 Dominica	99 Romania	162 Mauritania
36 Costa Rica	100 Saint Kitts and Nevis	163 Mali
37 USA	101 Moldova	164 Cameroon

We are supposedly the most powerful country in the world and yet we rank 37th in healthcare!? The current medical model of "Sick-Care" NOT health care, is broken. I approach the body with respect and awe. Working with the body, using symptoms as merely a sign that something else is wrong is critical. We focus on the cause of those symptoms...not the symptoms themselves. It would be like disconnecting the warning light in the dashboard of a car instead of adding fuel or oil or whatever the "warning signal" represented. Focus on the cause and the body can use its dynamic design to mount an attack on any condition out there.

Why You Should read This Book

This book gives you hope, if you, or someone you love, has been given the devastating diagnosis of cancer. In it you will discover how the body's immune system works and hear stories of many others that have tapped into the power of the body to heal itself. I have spoken at the Cancer Control Society's Cancer Convention on several occasions, constantly expanding my knowledge of how the body works.

"I had a grapefruit sized ovarian cyst while pregnant with Eli. MDs wanted me to terminate but Dr Bergman's treatment allowed for Eli to be born! Eli is happy and healthy now. I am blessed to have Dr Bergman and staff in my life."

-Suzy

"Doctors said Addison needed heart surgery as a baby. We avoided surgery because of chiropractic . She keeps growing and she had no heart failure. We've also been able to reduce her meds by two-thirds! The staff here is just like family."

-Nicole & Addison

“Old football injury resolved… Very pleased with results”

- Dean Torrence

“Meds almost did me in… I was very skeptical but was able to sit and stand without pain after treatment. I haven’t been sick for over a year following his health tips.”

- Mary

“My brother referred me...His results motivated me to come. I had severe scoliosis. On August3, 2009, Dr Bergman gave me back my life. Other chiropractors had said there wasn’t much they could do, but Dr Bergman fixed me. I can play with my Grandchildren again.

-Kathleen DeWyke

“My two younger brothers had had heart attacks and I was on my way. Under Dr Bergman’s care, my cholesterol dropped from 235 to 165 in only 6 weeks! Listen to him!”

-Fred

Table of Contents

INTRODUCTION

First off, thank you so much for investing in your health, because I've got to tell you, to take time out of your day just to learn something. This information is radically different than what you're going to learn from your doctor, and you're going to find out why, because a lot of this information's illegal. I know you're thinking, "Information is illegal?"

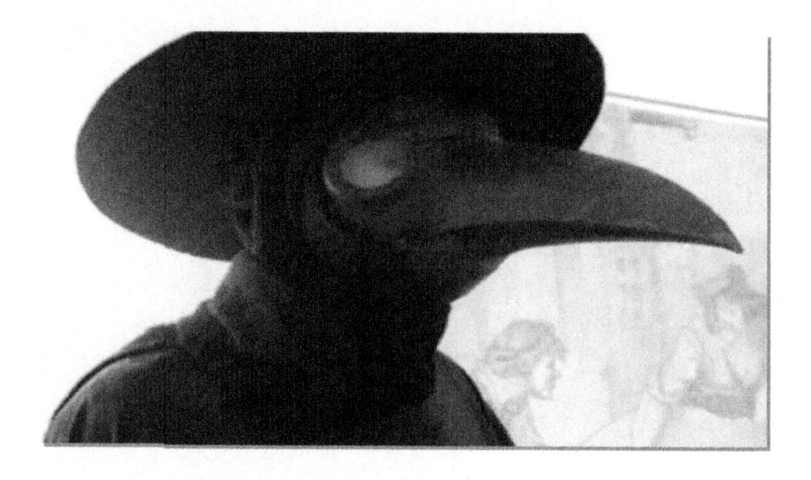

When we look at this, right now, if you're looking at that guy with the long nose, that's actually incredibly advanced technology for its time. At the time, we knew, without a doubt, that disease came from sin, evil spirits, and bad humors, bad air. In fact, that's why around swamps, we thought it had bad air. You know how to say 'bad air' in French? "Mal air". . . ria. See, we still use stupid terms like that. Of course, the red lenses means that spirits can't pass through red lenses. We look at this now, and we think that's really stupid, it's ignorant.

A lot of the therapies that we do nowadays are just as ignorant. When we looked at bleeding, you remember the practice of bleeding? It's what killed George Washington. That was started by the Egyptians, practiced thousands of years. It was practiced up until 1900. If you talked to the doctors in the late 1800's, late 1700's, 1600's, they would say, "Look, we have empirical data that this is what's been done for thousands of years. It's fantastically good. We know that the bad blood is in the dark ones, and the good blood is in the red ones, so we drain out the bad blood." This is stupid. OK?

Questions

The quality of your life depends on the quality of questions you ask, without a doubt, and I'm talking just in the next few years. We look at burning, which is radiation, and giving massive amounts of poison to the human body to kill fast-growing cells, and balancing the amount of poison without killing the healthy cells. This is going to be considered, in the next few years, incredibly stupid. This is modern technology. We're going to go over this, because it's not only harmful, but where's the scientific data for it? It's really similar to radiation. Let's look at actual facts. When we look at the *Kessler Report*, that survival rate hasn't changed in the last 55 to 60 years, but you're going to hear on the news that the five year survival rate is increasing. We're winning the war against cancer. Right, at five years. If you survive therapies after the diagnosis for five years and one day, you're considered cured. Raise your hand if you know somebody that had cancer. Keep your hand up if they had cancer with chemotherapy and it came back. There you go, about half. This is common. That group was considered cured, because they survived five years. It's working with the numbers. In actual fact, survival rates really haven't changed in over half a century.

95% OF CANCERS ARE PREVENTABLE

World health organizations say you can expect cancer rates to increase by over 50%. If we had a herd of water buffaloes and over half had cancer, would we go in there with surgery, chemotherapy, or radiation, or would we be looking for the cause? We'd be looking for the cause. Absolutely. Of course, I'm really not liking this thing. The people that wear the pink ribbons. Their heart is beautiful, their mind's in the right place. The organization is completely evil. We know that they spend less than one tenth of one percent of their budget on prevention. We know that 95 percent of all cancers are preventable. 95% of cancers are preventable. That's 95 percent of cancers are preventable. They're not looking into environmental causes. In 1970, when President Nixon declared the war on cancer, since then, cancer rates have increased over 90%. Are we winning the war or losing?

Losing the war. Massively. Since we want to have the appearance, because we need to keep generating the funds, because the American Cancer Society, I mean, this is one of the biggest moneymakers the planet has. It's not Run for the Cure, it's pinkwashing. I don't know if you remember a few years ago, but they got into deep trouble. Kentucky Fried Chicken, if you buy a bucket, they donate some money towards cancer research, even though there are massive cancer-causing agents in that bucket of chicken. It's almost humorous. I encourage you to watch the *Pink Ribbon* movie, because it's insane, what they do with the money, and how they pinkwash things. This is really not working.

ARE WE LIVING LONGER?

When we look at cancer rates among kids, as an adult with cancer, you could lie to yourself and say, 'Well, we're living longer. This is why slow-growing cancers are seen more.' That's not true. We're not living any longer than we were a hundred years ago. If you factor out infant mortality rate, we're about living the same length. If you look back at history, like when did Franklin die? When did Jefferson die? These men all passed in their mid-80's. But when we look at this, cancer rates among kids are increasing, and we don't know why. Why don't we know why, because we're not looking into it. If you're not going to look for something, you're not going to find it. We're not going to look at the environmental causes, we're not going to look at the vaccination rates, we're not going to look at the neuro-toxins and toxins that kids are exposed to. We're just seeing the rates go up.

POLITICS NOT HEALTH

When I was a kid, you didn't have bald kids on the counter. We had March of Dimes. We had kids with Muscular Dystrophy or we had kids with polio. Now, it's bald kids on the counter to raise money for, I don't know, the Saint Jude Hospital for Cancer. None of this stuff makes sense. When we look at this, Samuel Epstein says, we're not looking for the cure. In fact, I love the way he says, 'We're not dealing with a scientific problem. We're dealing with a political issue.' Because it is political. The income from cancer is tremendous. We're talking a $100 billion a year industry. When we look at this $100 billion a year industry, why are natural therapies suppressed? Or are they? Or is that a crazy conspiracy? Enough is enough. I'm going to tell you right now that's it's illegal. I can go in there, and if I was a medical doctor, I could say, "This orange will prevent scurvy." If I give you an orange in the purpose of a medical therapy to prevent scurvy, that's illegal, because the orange is not a medicine, even though, what did Hippocrates say? “Let food be your medicine, medicine be your food.” You think, as Americans, if you've read the Constitution and the Bill of Rights, that you're endowed by your creator with certain inalienable rights.

OUR CONSTITUTION

Well, not many people have read it, and it has been repealed, most of the aspects of the Constitution, but this one here. Back in 1979, Rutherford versus United States. There's a court case. This guy goes in there and exhausts his possibilities for health. He feels that as an American, the Constitution guarantees his right to choose whatever therapy he wants, so if he wants to choose Laetrile, if he wants to choose B17, if he wants to choose high-dose vitamin C in order to strengthen his immune system and fight a disease, as an American the U.S. Supreme Court says, "Yes, you have the right to choose that."

OK. They should be able to choose that. Bam! It's been taken away. The decision was reversed by the Food and Drug Administration. I know. What?! How can that be? How can the United States Supreme Court say that you, as an American, have a right, in a federal government institute, say, 'No, we have taken away the rights because, what? **What's the reasoning behind it?** They even say it here. "Well, it's the FDA's position, as they're the only ones in a position to approve whether it's good or bad. You don't have the intelligence, the intellect of the research data to prove therapies for yourself.' Is that insulting to anybody but me?

By gosh, I mean, if you give a child life, you're responsible for that child. You should be able to choose or not choose certain therapies. In this country, they're actually arresting parents for not getting chemotherapy on their child.

Even if it's proven there's no cancer.

ARE YOU FEEDING YOUR CANCER?

This is absolutely insane. We need to be aware that these types of laws are in force. That's actually stopping us. This is a really simple concept. If you feed cancer, it grows. If you starve it, it dies. There, that's the end of the lecture. No, but it's really that simple. When we look at this, the Fraud and Deception Association, I'm sorry, the FDA, Food and Drug Administration. They're approving certain toxic components that are actually feeding cancer. It's really a simple concept that we understand. When you look at this, this is out of the University of Irvine, if you had three hot dogs a week, your risk of brain cancer has increased tenfold. Being aware of this study, did the Food and Drug Administration close off all the supermarkets? We go in there, and we get the bologna and the hot dogs off of the shelves, or was it just, "No, that's an industry we don't mess with."

GENETICALLY MODIFIED ORGANISMS (GMO) AND FLUORIDE

When I was a kid, my bologna had a first name and a last name. But then again, when I was a kid, we didn't have genetically modified organisms, we didn't have bovine growth hormone, we didn't have multiple antibiotics and mold inside of the hot dogs. They weren't the healthiest animal, but they weren't poisonous. They weren't cancer-causing sticks like this.

When you look at the food labels, acrylamide, aspartame mono sodium glutamate and more!. We're literally choosing to poison ourselves. Cancer, by the way, is not a hair-loss disease. These bald kids are suffering from massive amounts of poisoning *from the only therapy that's approved by the government*. We have to take a stand. Dr. Dean Burk PhD spent thirty-four years with the national cancer institute. He was quoted as saying "In point of fact, fluoride causes more human cancer deaths and causes it faster than any other chemical." Who's going to vote for, let's see, let's see this, I know this is going to be a tough concept, but let's just try this. Mass-medication of the population without control of the dosage. Anybody? Anybody? OK. Welcome to fluoridation. It's absolutely stupid. Fluoride, a poison, inside of the system.

If you look at the original data from when fluoride was first done, it was all done by Alcoa Aluminum, because it's a byproduct of the aluminum industry. It's a byproduct of the fertilizer industry, which was a byproduct of the weapons industry. We have this toxic component that, oh, I don't know, we could pay millions of dollars to dispose of it, or we could get paid millions of dollars to dispose of it. As an industry, if you have no moral and ethics, what's better? Pay out a million dollars, or collect a million dollars?

Collect a million dollars.

But you have to get rid of your morals and ethics, because you're putting something toxic in the water supply. When you look at the history of fluoride, it's mind-boggling to think that fluoride is a toxic poison. It was used in German concentration camps, because it has a calming effect. It's a neurotoxin. This way, if you're drinking water, you're going to be a lot more calm. Obviously, I don't drink tap water. What's frustrating is, when you look at this, where's fluoride concentrated? Dole pineapple, Snapple, Coca Cola, sodas. They're using this fluoridated water in the packing process, and these are cancer-causing agents. You get somebody that wants to be healthy and they're going to use Rice Dreams, even though it has concentrated fluoride. They're trying to get away from dairy products. Or they're going to use Hanson's soda. Why? Because that's supposed to have fresh fruit in it. It's made with concentrated fluoride. This is not safe. The Fraud and Deception Association is approving this, but they're not approving oranges for cancer therapy. A seven ounce tube of toothpaste has enough fluoride in it to kill a small child. Should you be eliminating fluoride from your diet and from your children's diet, yes or yes?

Yeah, absolutely. Absolutely. And then when we look at this, this is one of the water filters we recommend Doulton Filters (www.Doulton.com). We give away about a water filter a month. This is a smaller version of the commercial version we have here. We have fluoride-free water here. Why? Because I want you to get better. I have fluoride-free water at my house. I have fluoride-free water at my boat. Why? Because I don't want to drink poison. I plan on being here for a while. This one, Doulton USA, a very reasonable filter, and it only costs around $217 for around 300 liters, so it's very, very reasonable.

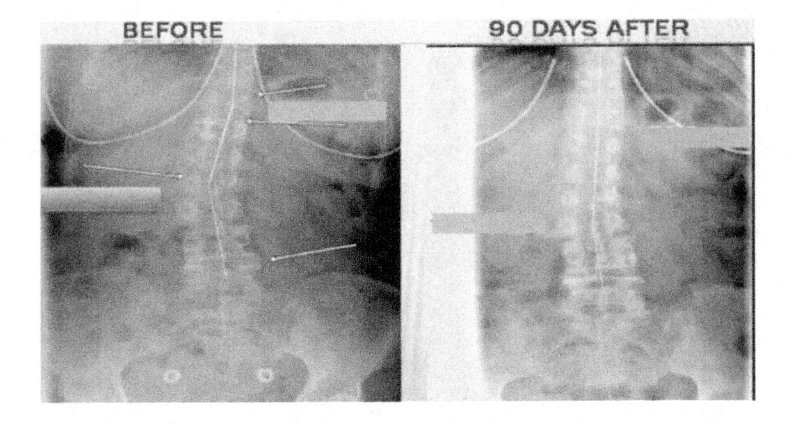

This patient here, when you look at it, that's the X-ray. In this modern therapy, is she given healthy nutrition? No. Depression, fatigue fibromyalgia syndrome. She was given multiple medications. Understand, in the old days, we used to call it 'patent medicine.' That means, in order to produce a drug, it had to be something that's never been seen in the human body, it's never been seen on the planet, so it's patentable, and this is every medication around there.

RISKS OF MEDICATIONS

Have you ever heard of drug called 'acetaminophen'?

What's it's brand name? Starts with a "T"?

Tylenol! Do you know how that works? Shake your head.

No. Because neither do they. It says, "mechanism of action is unknown." We don't know. Have you seen the antidepressants, like Wellbutrin, Prozac, Depakote, Elavil? They're called 'selective serotonin reuptake inhibitors." Do you know how those work?

No. Neither do they. In clinical pharmacology, we don't know. We haven't a clue at how they work. In fact, when you look at most actions, or pharmaceutical products, they're only going to do two things. They're either going to poison an enzyme or block a receptor site in a cell. Every medication you're prescribed is going to change a metabolic process. When you get depression, fatigue, and fibromyalgia syndrome, you're talking antidepressants, antacids, sleep medications, pain relievers, muscle relaxants. This is modern society. I'm thinking back at that guy with the long nose. This is absolute foolishness. Remember, we're looking at a population where 50 percent of us has cancer. What's the number one therapy recommended by doctors to screen for cancer?

MAMMOGRAMS

Mammograms, unless you're looking at this. Screening for breast cancer with mammograms is unjustified.

> The authors own words say it best: "Screening for breast cancer with mammography is unjustified." They also found that it causes six times more deaths than it prevents (Lancet 2000; 355: 129-134)

This is the Lancet, European medical journal. OK. Unjustified. When you look at this one, it causes six times more cancer than they prevent. Mammograms worthless overall breast exam. Hand palpating is much better than mammograms. For half a million women, for every one woman that mammograms help, ten are harmed. Were you aware of this? OK. What's the only therapy approved? What's wild is, this is the big push to get you into the system, to find some type of problem so that you get, literally, all the therapies that are in the system. First off, you're going to get a biopsy, then, you're going to get a couple of consultations. If they find any abnormal cell growth, they can put you on some chemical therapy. This is a huge rush. However, when we look at this, ten times the amount of women have heart disease. So why isn't there a great push for cleaning arteries? This is the moneymaker.

Dr Lorraine Day

This gal is a rebel. If you like heroes, this is one of my favorites. Her name is Dr. Lorraine Day, DrDay.com. I found her about 14-15 years ago, back when we had cassettes. They were small little square things. They had a little reel to reel in them. They were really cool.

She was Head of Orthopedic Surgery at San Francisco Memorial…a brilliant gal. She develops breast cancer. Not just breast cancer. It metastasized to her chest wall and lung. This is really dangerous. She cures herself using no mastectomy, no chemotherapy, no radiation.

Cures herself.

I find this interesting, so I call her up and I get the 12 cassettes. The first cassette is on conspiracy therapies. Second cassette's on conspiracy therapies. Third cassette's on how the medical industry needs to promote cancer. I'm going, "Come on, man! I've got patients. I can't sit here through all these 12 tapes. Just show me the herb. I just want to tell somebody." Because I'm not a conspiracy theorist.

Her Secret

Tape 11, still, she's talking about the medical conspiracy. Finally, she gets to tape 12 and she tells me the secret. You ready?

"If man makes it, don't eat it. Attitude of gratitude. Deep sleep is really important."

OK. Strengthen the immune system, don't poison yourself. Wow! Can it be that simple? Can human beings actually cure themselves? Yeah, absolutely.

Cancer Healing Resources

I encourage you to look at some of the websites, because these therapies are illegal in this country. Burzynski's clinic (www.Burzynkiclinic.com) developed his own antineoplasm therapy, where he has been curing breast cancer, brain cancer, I mean, real hard cancers. He developed his own therapy, and he's been practicing this for about 30 years, and they just recently, I think just in the last couple of weeks, took his ability to heal people. A couple of great videos on him.

Gerson Therapy (gerson.org/gerpress/get-started/) has been curing and reversing diseases and chronic diseases and cancer for about 80 years. That's a phenomenal website for research, and it's absolutely incredible. I will even send you a downloadable PDF summary of what to look for, so you don't even need to write it down. Just call, TOLL FREE 1-866-603-3995 and enter pin #: 94500 Follow the instructions and you will receive a link via email to the handout and a bonus video.

PROSTATE CANCER

Then we look at prostate. I've got so many patients that come here and say, "Oh, my husband's PSA is elevated!" PSA stands for "prostate specific antigen", which is kind of a misnomer, because it's not really specific to the prostate. It's really high in women who have breast cancer and who are recovered from, and it's completely inaccurate. Dr. Stamey developed the test. I love this quote, from him in the Journal of the National Cancer Institute: 'I removed a few hundred prostates I wish I hadn't.'

If you've had your prostate removed, you're talking many, many, many problems. Dysfunctions, bowel and bladder control problems. I have a patient now, he's in his early 70's, and he was told when he was 60, "Your PSA is elevated. We've got to take the prostate out." He said, "Yeah, I want life. OK. I'll lose a lot of function, but take it out. I'm strong. Do the aggressive therapy." They take it out. Ten years go by. His PSA goes back up. He goes into the oncologist and he says, "Look, you said if I had it removed, I wouldn't have a problem. Why is the PSA going up? Why do I have cancer now?" They said, "Well, sometimes it just reoccurs. We're going to get you on some high-dose chemotherapy."

There's even a book by Dr. Larry Clapp on how to cure prostate cancer. It's very simple. Don't poison yourself, get high-dose vegetables, and your prostate will shrink, and then you've got to take care of the nerves that supply the pelvic area. This is insanity, that they're just going to take a random blood test, say that you have something, and remove it. It's just completely not consistent with science.

WHY DO HALF OF AMERICANS HAVE CANCER?

Then we come up with the big one. Why does 50% of our population have it? There's epigenetic control. If you understand genes, you can control gene expression. You can control your ability to fight cancer, or your ability to cause cancer. Genetic expression is everything. First off, cancer is not genetic. Cancer is not genetic. Cancer is not genetic. What did I just say?

Cancer is not genetic.

I want to make sure. Because, when you view the TV, they say, "Oh, cancer is genetic, heart disease is genetic. If your mom had breast cancer…" They're doing prophylactic breast removals, and that is just sick! Save the breast, baby! No, but you can't do that stuff. It's stupid, OK? If cancer's not genetic, there's a control above the genes. It's called 'genetic expression.'

Blue eyes don't change color. That's genetic. But if you have something that works great for 20 or 30 or 40 years, and then all of a a sudden you develop breast cancer or high blood pressure or diabetes, that's genetic expression. So there's a control above the genes, and we know this.

Dr. Bruce Lipton has been studying it for years. Multiple books have been written on it. What's interesting now though is, we now know that medications have an epigenetic control. If you look at this list here, you're looking at everything, from anti-inflammatories, this is going to be non-steroidal anti-inflammatories, blood pressure drugs, cholesterol drugs, anti-depression drugs, sleep drugs. Does this mean every medication has an epigenetic control? Yes or yes? This means every medication which is a patentable drug, which is something that's foreign to your body that's never been seen on the planet, created by a chemist, is going to have a negative effect on your body. Is that clear?

This means when you watch the stupid commercials that say, "Look, don't you want to be running through this field of flowers and be happy if you're sad? However, the side-effects are increased leukemia. Tell your doctor if you've ever had tuberculosis. If your doctor thinks this is right for you, make sure you don't have any bleeding behind the eyes or high blood pressure." They go on for seven minutes like this. We can't do this. We've got to take the blinders off. What's worse about this, and this is one of the most brilliant quotes I've ever seen: "Consequences for modern medicine are profound, since it would imply that our current understanding of pharmacology is an oversimplification." No kidding. This solves pain, but it'll cause cancer. This thing here will get you to sleep, but you're going to be depressed. This anti-depressant will cause you to go insane and maybe want you to shoot somebody. OK. We're numbed into this. Thank God we're drinking the fluoride, otherwise people would be upset. I didn't just say that, did I?

CASE STUDY

OK. This is a typical patient. I changed her name to Amy. She's diagnosed with lupus. Think of this. This is modern medicine. Lupus is an incurable, auto-immune disorder. Eight years old, she comes and she says, "Yeah, I was perfectly healthy." Right, OK. Born natural at home or in a hospital? She was born in a hospital. You can't have a natural birth in the hospital, by the way. It's impossible. She's eight years old. She developed this rash and joint pain after playing in the sandbox, in a brand new sandbox. They said, "Were there other kids playing in the sandbox?" She said, "Yeah." I said, "Did everybody get the same rash?" "No." I said, "Well, why did you get this rash?" "I don't know." She looked at me, because the doctors had told her, "Since you got the rash after playing in the sand, it was probably the sand." I'm thinking, no. Then, let's look at her history. Her mom was given Pitocin. This is a drug from a cow that interrupts the dance during the birth process and causes massive uterine contractions, injuring the child's neck. It hurt the mom so much they gave her an epidural so that she wouldn't feel the pain. So, birth trauma. With birth trauma, she had ear infections. We know now that antibiotics don't help with ear infections, but what was she prescribed?

Antibiotics. You know this. That causes leaky gut, causes large proteins to get in there, and weakens the immune system, causes brain damage. Also, fully, vaccinated. She's going to get 81 shots before the age of 6. OK. Does that sound like a lot?

2026

It is a lot. It's completely unusual. Nobody's ever experimented like that. There's only one animal study that was done in 2008 in Pittsburgh University and 100% of the primates that got that developed neurological conditions similar to those. If anybody says that vaccines aren't causing neurological damage or autism, just say 2026 to them. 2026 is the year that the number of kids with autism will outnumber the kids without autism.

No, you don't need to worry. It's going to be fixed this year.

No, it is. It is. Don't think I'm kidding here. See, they're going to change the diagnostics. We're going to have the same number of sick kids. It just won't be labeled as autism. Phew! Boy, that was close. That was an epidemic that almost got us. The same number of brain-damaged people will be here, but we're going to label it different, so this way, as long as you're drinking the fluoride, you won't worry.

This little kid with joint pain and rash went to 15 different doctors. 15! They flew down from San Francisco and they're saying, "Hey, look, 15 different doctors. Bam! This is the definitive diagnosis." I said, "Well, I don't agree with it." They gave her some steroid cream and they said, "OK. What can you do?" Their relatives had had some miracles, so they said, "Hey, go see this chiropractor in Huntington Beach."

They fly down and I say, "Look, you're taking neurotoxins, you've got multiple neurotoxins injected in you, your gut is horrible, you've got pressure on the brain stem here. We're going to get you adjusted and change your diet."

She was only down here for three days. We got her a couple of adjustments. She goes back home, I get a call, about a month later. She says, "Oh my gosh! Her joint pain's better. She doesn't have the rash. She's feeling better. The entire family went on the diet. They're feeling great. She doesn't have it anymore." Aaaah! The human body's a miracle.

Look for the Cause

This is insanity. This is modern medical care. You don't have one doctor that ties it all in unless they're a chiropractor. You've got the neurologist that says, "Well, yeah, you've got a pinched nerve radiating pain down here." I'm doing another book, and our last book just became a bestseller, on arthritis reversal. This other book's on fibromyalgia. I looked up the definitive expert on fibromyalgia, who happened to be the head of California university. The guy is saying, "Well, joint pain, this drug is effective. This pain, this drug is effective."

They're saying, "Nine out of ten fibromyalgia had some kind of trauma before the onset of it." I'm going, "Look for the trauma!" They can't find it. Look for the actual reason for it. The gastroenterologist is skilled in looking at diseases of the digestive tract. He's not taught nutrition! The pulmonologist is not taught that the nerves control the lungs, that asthma is a problem with the nervous system, the smooth muscle control. He has to talk to the neurologist, but the neurologist doesn't know anything. The neurotransmitters that are produced in the gut can affect the autonomic nervous system. Heck, they're all looking at these different diseases. Then you get the dermatologist. Rashes, a skin problem, just like, what is it, chicken pox? Is chicken pox a skin disease?

No. That's the body exuding toxins out of the system. It's a systemic disorder. Every one of these doctors needs to be acquainted with the systemic system, that the body is in one system, that has to function correctly.

A Pharmacy on Every Corner

Statins cause cancer. Why? Because statins lower cholesterol. Cholesterol is the most complex molecule you've got. It's the precursor to everything your adrenal glands make. Your adrenal glands produce every glucocorticid steroid, medicocorticoid steroid, sex hormone, and they're reducing it? With a drug? How ignorant! My gosh, they should all be wearing hats like that, so we could recognize them. Take off the white jacket, start wearing this if you're going to prescribe a drug. Come on, guys, that's ridonkulous.

Antibiotics, nonsteroidal anti-inflammatories. How many kids are given antibiotics for ear infections that aren't required? How many kids are given Tylenol to reduce a fever, which is absolutely insane? When we look at this, we're seeing a massive rise of Non-Hodgkin's lymphoma. Why? Because these medications should not be used in human beings. Why? Because they're not natural in human beings. We don't know the effects. How does Tylenol work? We don't know. We know that most antibiotics are poisonous mold. That's just not effective. This is one of the scams. Because we are drinking, we're not going to remember this, but back before 2002, I live about a mile and a half away from here. I pass seven pharmacies on the way. Seven pharmacies. Where my boat is, there's one street that has absolutely no pharmacies on it. It's called Pacific Avenue. I love driving on it. There's a bar on every third corner, but there's not one pharmacy.

Yeah, I know, it's really kind of fun. It's like, "No CVS. I like this". When you go by it, in CVS, there's flu shot, flu shot, flu shot. There used to be a flu season. Nope, that's discounted. You drink the fluoride, you're not going to remember it. Now, it's all year long. What's wild is, in 2002, they said, every healthy American over 50. Before, it was only sick people. Then, 2002, they added babies, 6 months to 23 months. There's no study that shows that it's safe. These are flu shots. Then, 2006, healthy children up to 5, so 6 months to 5 years old now. Damn! OK. We're getting this under the umbrella. You're seeing this massive increase in vaccinations. Vaccinations have neurotoxins in there. They actually cause the body to attack itself. Where was the damage? Where was the danger? 300 million Americans, this is what increase of this medication use. Wait a second. That means there were less than 2000 people dying? Where was the panic? I think there's 730 lightning strikes in America, people struck my lightning. So there are more people being struck by lightining than dying of the flu? Can you see this? Where's the panic? The panic is totally, totally manufactured. Luckily, 2007, 2008, 2009, Homeland Security stepped in. Yes, they're now a medical facility.

They said that since terrorists in Afghanistan can build a virus that could infect all 300 million Americans that now all of the manufacturing companies that produced a flu shot are exempt from any damage, so if you get Guillain-Barre, if you get autism, if you get neurological damage, if you get cancer, which are all side effects of the shots. It says it on the package.

It says it on the package before you inject yourself, you can't sue them since 2009.

2010 was the greatest year for the CDC. That's the year that annual flu shots for everyone, from six months old till death, every year, you get a shot, no matter what. This is an experiment if you want to opt in for, you are drinking the fluoride. I'd recommend not, and let the other people take the shot, and apartments will be cheaper, because there'll be more available.

This is insane. This is absolutely a crazy medical procedure that's approved for everyone. We know vaccines can cause molecular mimicry. Every time you get a shot, your body produces antibodies. If your body produces antibodies that are supposed to be towards that virus or bug or bacteria or neurotoxins, if it doesn't produce it, it can produce so many antibodies that they'll attack certain things. If they attack the nervous system, it'll be multiple sclerosis. Attack the joints, rheumatoid arthritis, scleroderma. These are autoimmune disorders caused by vaccinations.

When I get a patient in here who's got major toxic effects, like that kid with lupus, I say, "Are they fully vaccinated or modified vaccine schedule?" Luckily, parents are looking into this, because that's just insanity. They even know that it's linked to vaccinations, but they're not going to check it. Why does 50% of our population have cancer? Why does 50% of our population have cancer? Our medical therapies and our food that's approved for human consumption, which isn't food.

This gal, just darling. She comes in, five years old, her parents say, "She can't sleep. She gets up at 2 or 3 o'clock in the morning." What does that sound like? It sounds like she's in this fight-or-flight state, right? Sure enough, guess what happened. Hospital birth. Do you think that there was some trauma there? More than likely. Extreme skin sensitivity, poor digestion. This means fully vaccinated, so she has leaky gut syndrome, she has major neurological damage. She comes in here, we get her adjusted. She slept the first night. Then we start her on healthy nutrition. She's doing incredibly well now, incredibly well. What's frustrating is that she would be just choked off in this medical world. Sunlight decreases breast cancer. If you look at where the equator is, there's very little to no breast cancer around the equator. The further away from the equator, larger amounts of breast cancer. If you look at lung cancer of women in Canada, 60% never smoked, but there's less vitamin D.

In this country, what are the doctors saying? "Avoid the sun! Put the sunblock on!'"However, there's no scientific data that supports that that's healthy for you. It's absolutely insane. Breast cancer, colon cancer, rectal cancer. Prostate, OK. We have to keep it. It's vital for us. Vitamin E, so we're looking at nuts, seeds, selenium, Omega-3s. This is just all healthy food of normal human consumption. If you're taking burgers, if you're taking the hot dogs, that's a huge Omega 6 to 3 ratio. We need a 1 to 1. Since our diet is horrible, we need to have Omega-3 supplements. We have an algae-based one I really recommend. We need ground flax seeds, daily vegetables. It sounds too simple, that you could just change your diet, not poison yourself, eliminate medications, and your body will fight cancer. Doesn't it sound too simple? Well, it's true. This is the battle that goes on in your body.

The Immune System

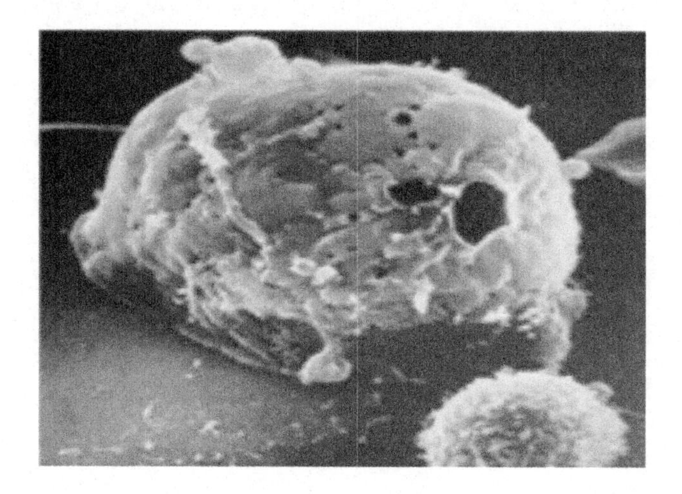

This right here is a large, ugly cancer cell. That's an immune system cell. It's called a "killer cell". It's actually called a "natural killer cell." It goes in and attaches to a cell, destroys the cell, leaving this in its matrix, and it's ready to do battle again. This battle occurs at least 10 thousand times a day. Your body produces a billion cells a day. I have cancer in my body. It's never going to be effective in taking over my life. Why? Because I've got an immune system. I don't want to impress you. I'm made in the image and likeness of God. He's probably in better shape than me. You are too. Utilize the natural power inside of your body to initiate this battle, because that's what it does. I mean, right here, you can see that's a reverse curve in the neck. Do you think that knowing that the breathing muscle, the diaphragm, the phrenic nerve that supplies the diaphragm, comes out of the base of the neck. Do you think if you have a reversal of the curve, that that diaphragm won't function well?

OK. Just for the heck of it. Try it. Take a deep breath in. Blow it out. You see the carbon monoxide go out?..That's acid. You're losing acid, so you have healthy breathing function. You're going to have less cancer rates. Why am I so obsessive about making sure that the neck has a healthy arc in it? Because it's vital. It's called 'the arc of life'.

THERMOGRAPHY

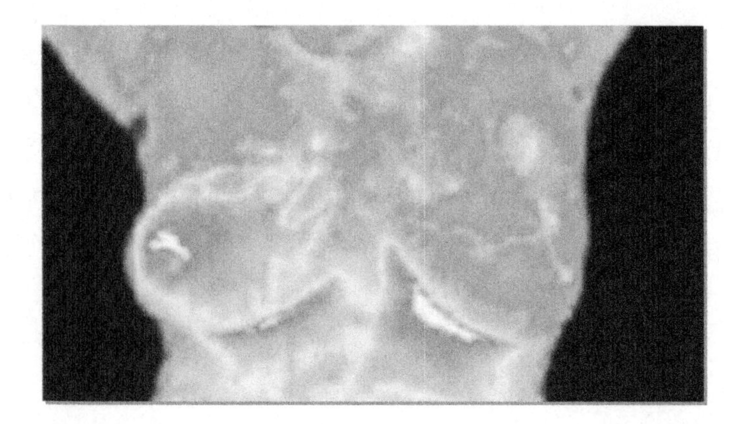

Thermography? This one, again, is not approved by the Fraud and Deception Association, because it's effective. A mammogram can identify a lump the size of a head of a pin, which means it's been growing nine years. Thermography can identify abnormal cell growth within three months. If you more advanced technology with less toxins, this is fantastic, because if you identify abnormal cell growth like that, you can change your diet, change your therapies, increase your immune system, and do another check in 90 days, and you can see it different. The human body is amazing.

When we look at this, I mean, God bless lipstick. There's nothing that looks prettier than makeup. However, it's got toxic components in it, so make sure that ev[illegible] the makeup that girls wear, or guys, I can't be a judge, I mean, in my year, only girls wore lipstick contains lead, contains heavy metal. When you're getting that, look at the label. One of the most frustrating things, when you see that *Pink Ribbon* movie is, a lot of those walks are sponsored by Revlon. Revlon contains cancer causing products, and they're sponsoring the cancer walk. Do they come right out and say, 'Hey, look, our products cause cancer, so we're going to go in and try and help defeat the cancer that we're causing'? No. That's not effective.

This guy, Dr. Simoncini (www.curenaturalicancro.com), he's also one of the sites on here. He had a theory that cancer is a fungus. You've got to figure, for seven years, they haven't been able to find a pathogenic cause of cancer. This means they're looking for the virus, they're looking for the bacteria, they're looking for the bug, the pathogen, the thing that causes it. However, what they found, they can't find it. This guy is a pediatric oncologist. Every time he removes a cancerous tumor, it's white, so he's thinking, maybe it's fungus. He goes in there and he does a sodium bicarbonate drip. Anybody know what sodium bicarbonate is?

Baking soda. You're right, so you can't get a patent on it. Ah, bummer! Let's use it anyway. He is Italian, so he says, "Why not? Let's try it." He does it. He'll hook it up to an artery that supplies the area, and you're seeing brain tumors shrink, lung tumor shrink. You're seeing this one here, uterine tumor, shrink. OK. He's thinking, "Wow! Alkalinizing the system locally in that area shrinks tumors. I have one of the cures for cancer." That's pretty cool, huh? Yeah, I think they took his medical license away. I'm not sure. Because the medical conglomerate, the medical mafia, we can call it, is very, very well and happy in Europe, just like it is in our country. Our country, it's a little bit more aggressive.

Then when we look at this, hydrogen peroxide therapy. This is massive amounts of oxygen in a cell, and your cells actually secrete something similar to this to knock out cancer. Multiple books on hydrogen peroxide therapy. Multiple, multiple, multiple books. They're doing IV drips in some countries, they're taking it orally in some countries. Just for fun, I look at the American Cancer Society. It states there's no scientific evidence that hydrogen peroxide is a safe or useful cancer treatment and advises cancers to remain in the care of qualified doctors who use proven methods of treatment. Proven methods of treatment. There hasn't been a change in death rates in over 60 years. Proven? The only thing that's proven is stuff that the Fraud and Deception Association approves of? No. Health revolution is now. These guys, this is actual doctors that are curing cancer. Run from the cure.

I think it's Rick Simpson's story (www.youtube.com/user/chrychek). This guy developed skin cancer in Canada, went online, found that you can make an oil from the cannabis plant, and he cured cancer, and then he helped his friend cure lung cancer with it. Dr. Lorraine Day. Gerson therapy. Hoxsey therapy. Laetrile. B17. We're coming up to the fruit season. When you guys get a peach pit or an apricot kernel, split it open, eat the thing on the inside. It' [illegible] t's loaded with B17. It's fantastic. Just look at B17. There's multiple studies on this. It's called Laetrile in some countries. It reverses cancer. This is incredible.

Knockout, Suzanne Somers. I read that book. I think we've got it in our lending library. She goes into a standard oncologist, and then she goes into Dr. Gonzalez in New York, who's doing the William Kelley method (educate-yourself.org/cancer/kellysmetabolictherapy.shtml). William Kelly method's very effective on pancreatic and liver cancer. She calls up Dr. Gonzalez and says, 'Hey, do you have ten names of ten people that survived your therapy ten years? Liver and pancreatic?' He said, 'Sure, give me a minute. I'll give you a call back with their numbers. You can call them.'

He does, gives her back the numbers of people. She calls her oncologist and says, "Hey, Doc, do you have ten people that have survived ten years with your therapy, the chemotherapy, the radiation?"

"Ten years? Dude, we're lucky to get them ten months!"

I'm speaking at the Cancer Control Society this coming September. It's every Labor Day Weekend in Universal Studios. They haven't told me what I'm speaking on, but it's more than likely going to be on medications causing cancer. This is just brilliant. These are proven cancer therapies. I'm sorry, not approved, just proven. They work. OK. Gerson theory. B17. B6. Multiple studies on B6. Burzynski. Hopefully he can move across to Mexico and set up a nice clinic. Eliminate toxins. The rave diet. We've got a couple of videotapes on the RAVE diet. Simoncini. Day. Avoid pharmaceuticals and avoid toxins. It's really, really that simple.

Disease Risk Asessment Checklist

We've got to start approaching people with respect. This is food. This is part of the secret formula. Dr. Lorraine Day treated and successfully eliminated cancer. If man makes it, you don't eat it. If it grows, you do. This is actually really good stuff to eat.

You need these five points.

You need to get your nervous system checked for subluxation.

You need to have regular exercise, and this is just to detox your body. Sedentary lifestyle is going to cause toxic buildup.

You need to have healthy nutrition.

You need to have sufficient rest.

You need prayer and meditation.

Where do you think I got these five points? It's from that Dr. Day. This is literally the same thing that you can cure cancer with.

JOIN THE OWNERS-GUIDE FAMILY

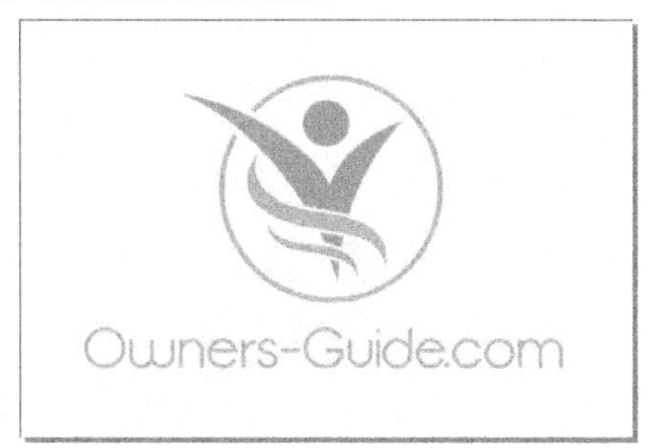

Earlier this year we created a membership site to keep people informed of the dangers of the current medical model and how to live an optimal life. We have members from all across the world from Australia to Ireland and Connecticut to Texas. This site offers videos, downloadable handouts, powerpoint slides, audio versions in MP3, a members only facebook group to share personal health challenges and victories and the latest data on future trips and speaking engagements we are planning. Go to www.owners-guide.com/membership-account/membership-levels for more information.

Connect with Dr Bergman

Thank you so much fro taking the time to read this book. I'm excited for you to start your path to optimal health using this new knowledge. Your eyes have been opened. The rest is up to you.

If you have any questions of any kind, feel free to contact me at info@owners-guide.com

You can follow me on Twitter: @johnbchiro

You can check out my membership site for the latest updates here: Owners-Guide.com

All memberships start with a 7 day FREE trial.

I'm wishing you the very best of health, happiness and LIFE!

Here's to you!

Dr. John Bergman

About the Author

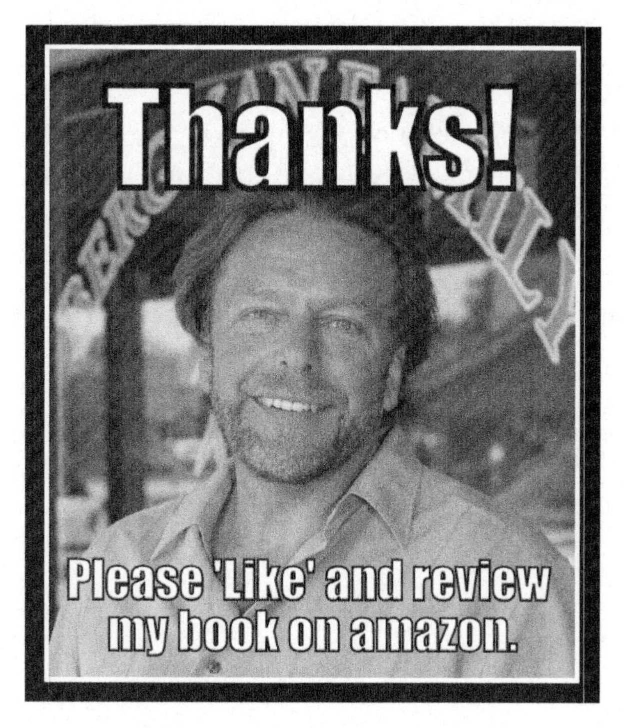

I was launched into chiropractic by a devastating accident that nearly ended my life. At 30 years old, I was a hard working single dad when I was hit by a speeding car that left me with 2 fractured legs, a fractured skull and chest, bruised liver and heart. Thankfully, I received the finest medical care that saved my life. However after 4 knee surgeries and multiple medications, I knew that surgeries and drugs were not the answer to regaining health.

Disillusioned by the modern symptom based mechanistic health care system, I began a quest to find a vitalistic based healthcare model to regain my health. I became an instructor at Cleveland Chiropractic College in Los

Angeles Specializing in Human Anatomy, Physiology, Biomechanics and multiple Chiropractic Techniques.

I developed my own techniques and have an extensive knowledge of human anatomy and human physiology that few can match. My unique approach has led to many successes, in even the most challenging cases.

I am the #1 Best Selling Author of How to Reverse Arthritis Naturally and How to Recover from Fibromyalgia: Real Solutions for a Real Problem. My latest work, *How to Correct High Blood Pressure Without Medications*, is scheduled for release in early Fall 2013.

To learn more about me and other books, speaking engagements and videos go to:

John Bergman's Author Page

www.amazon.com/-/e/B00BPB2OSO

ONE LAST THING

Thanks for reading! If you enjoyed this book or found it useful, I'd be very grateful if you'd post a short review on Amazon. Your support really does make a difference and I read all the reviews personally so I can get your feedback and make this and future books even better.

If you'd like to leave a review then all you have to do is click the review link on this book's page on Amazon here:

http://www.amazon.com/review/create-review

Thanks again for your support!

Dr John Bergman

Printed in Great Britain
by Amazon